The Monster Inside of Me:

Life with Borderline Personality Disorder

Brooke Price

Cover Art By:

Mr. Michael Tolleson

This book is dedicated to

Mrs. Andrea Krouse.

Thanks for the inspiration and your true friendship.

And to

Mr. Michael Tolleson.

Thank you for your kindness and your talent. The use of your painting for the cover made this book perfect. You are a true friend.

Also from Brooke Price

Living Through Autism's Eyes:

My Journey with My Son

Melting Down Meltdowns:

When a Tantrum isn't a Tantrum

Beautiful Disasters:

A Look Inside of Bipolar Disorder

Redefining Normal:

A Real World Guide to Raising an Autistic Child

Painting the Spectrum Gold:

Advancements in Autism

1

Borderline Personality Disorder (BPD) is an extremely serious mental illness affecting approximately 1 in 50 adults, or 2% of the United States population. (Statistics about Borderline Personality Disorder, 2015) It is like a little monster inside of us, waiting to pounce. At this time, there is a much-needed calling for advocacy for this ostensibly invisible illness, mostly because so little is known about Borderline Personality Disorder. Much of what is known is marginalized and made light of until it seems to be nothing more than an extreme mood had by an individual who seems immature. Nothing could be farther from the truth though. Having an immaturity of emotions due to a clinical diagnosis is different than being overall immature in life. Primarily emotional instability, difficulties in regulating behavior and interpersonal relationships are the essential features of BPD. (Korkeila J, 2015) This monster inside of me is so much more though.

The DSM, Fourth Edition, Text Revision (DSM-IV-TR) states that a person must show an "enduring pattern" of at least five of the following symptoms in order to be diagnosed BPD:

-Extreme reactions—including panic, depression, rage, or frantic actions—to abandonment, whether real or perceived

-A pattern of intense and stormy relationships with family, friends, and loved ones, often veering from extreme closeness and love (idealization) to extreme dislike or anger (devaluation)

-Distorted and unstable self-image or sense of self, which can result in sudden changes in feelings, opinions, values, or plans and goals for the future (such as school or career choices)

-Impulsive and often dangerous behaviors, such as spending sprees, unsafe sex, substance abuse, reckless driving, and binge eating

-Recurring suicidal behaviors or threats or self-harming behavior, such as cutting

-Intense and highly changeable moods, with each episode lasting from a few hours to a few days

-Chronic feelings of emptiness and/or boredom

-Inappropriate, intense anger or problems controlling anger

-Having stress-related paranoid thoughts or severe dissociative symptoms, such as feeling cut off from oneself, observing oneself from outside the body, or losing touch with reality. (Borderline Personality Disorder, n.d.)

Living with this disorder isn't effortless. It seems to either leave you with a feeling of almost complete indifference in everything you do and say or leaves you with a feeling of constant turmoil over every choice you make. There seems to be little variation in the general feeling based on interviews and other research done. This is often accompanied by bouts of extreme rage sat off by almost anything. Often it is triggered by a confusion of emotions or an overwhelming amount of said emotions. This is often caused by things such as feeling anger instead of embarrassment, shame/humiliation instead of embarrassment, or guilt instead of joy.

Some of us also have an issue with how mad we get whenever we do feel rage. Some of us even report blackouts, completely losing track of pieces of time. One second we can be mad and the next second have turned off. We become almost "another person," saying and doing things we'd ordinarily never do or say. Then there can also be bouts of depression. The depression is often marked with bouts of self-harm and suicidal thoughts; as well as many other impulsive behaviors that can be experienced simultaneously by a person with BPD.

When faced with the question as to which symptom was the worse I turned to an online support group for my answers. I polled the group based on their experiences with the symptoms listed in the DSM-IV-TR. When polled the tight knit support group of sufferers listed highly changeable moods and an unstable sense of self as the two symptoms of this disorder that affects them the most. I must agree.

Highly changeable moods, splitting, and an unstable sense of self are the symptoms that affect me the most daily when dealing with this monster.

Through this book, I will break down some of these symptoms by chapter, in order to give you a better view of Borderline Personality Disorder as seen through our eyes. I will give viewpoints from other sufferers, and from myself. I will offer statistics and a one of a kind look into what it is like for the partner of someone with this disorder, as well. So, sit back and relax, you are about to enter a little known or understood world.

2

The DSM-IV-TR lists 6 different personality disorder types. These disorders being:

-Borderline Personality Disorder

-Obsessive-Compulsive Personality Disorder

-Avoidant Personality Disorder

-Schizotypal Personality Disorder

-Antisocial Personality Disorder

-Narcissistic Personality Disorder.

(Association, 2013)

Yes, BPD is listed with Schizotypal disorders.

Extreme reactions—including panic, depression, rage, or frantic actions—to abandonment, whether real or perceived (Borderline Personality Disorder, n.d.) seems to be one of the number one symptoms suffered by individuals with BPD. It's the first symptom listed by the DSM-IV-TR and the first one mentioned by every sufferer I personally speak too. Specifically, intense rage, which is listed as a symptom by itself.

Often when reacting in an extreme fashion the BPD sufferer has little recollection of what caused them to react the way they did. This has a strong correlation to anger, as seen in the interviews I have done. We remember being mad and that there was a fight but often the details become fuzzy afterward. This is not an excuse; it is a fact. There are even times when the Borderline sufferer has no recollection that they were more than mad, that they were enraged.

The Borderline tends to "turn-off" becoming almost a different type of person. No, they are not clinically a different person but the overload of extreme emotions pushes us into acting in a manner that is that of a different person all together. We are not ourselves. We may say things or do things that we'd never do otherwise.

Sometimes if you ask the BPD sufferer or their loved ones about this they will tell you that the individual is a different person even though clinically that is not the case. This is also not the case with every Borderline. Some do not feel like a different person when they "turn-off," they simply can't remember what occurred clearly. Whenever I "turn-off" I consider myself a completely different person whose actions I am responsible for.

The responsibility of the actions of a Borderline have been one of the most highlighted points, nationally, of this disorder. Most of the symptoms of BPD are little known; however, the potential danger of a Borderline was thrusted into the national spotlight with trials such as the Jodi Arias trial. For those of you that do not know, Jodi Arias is the young woman from California that stabbed her former lover (Mr. Travis Alexander) 27 times, shot him in the head, and then slit his throat ear to ear in Mesa, AZ.

Following these actions Ms. Arias went to great lengths to cover her tracks. During her trial, she claimed to not remember anything. She later recanted, stating she remembered what she had done but that it was fuzzy. She manipulated the system in every way she could, including trying to manipulate guards. For the longest time, she went on record claiming that she was never at Mr. Alexander's house that night. Later she claimed that other people broke in and killed him, but she got away.

During her first trial, she claimed that Mr. Alexander attacked her. She stuck with that story for quite some time. The gun used in the crime was never recovered, the knife and pictures of the crime while it was taking place were. Ms. Arias never went on record with any memory of what she did with the gun. During her first of two trials, she was diagnosed with BPD. None the less she was sentenced to life in prison without the possibility of parole.

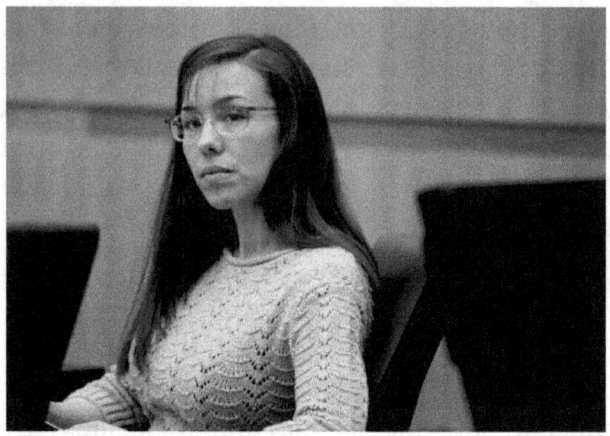
Figure 2 Jodi Arias during her first trial. Picture Courtesy of Youtube.com

This crime, fueled with the hallmarks of BPD's extreme reactions of rage and panic, was a prime example of debate on whether Borderlines should be held accountable for their actions. America's and the world's television sets were flooded with scenes of protesters on both sides of the situation, all having sympathy for Mr. Alexander's family. Some also feeling that a person with such an obvious mental issue shouldn't be held accountable for their actions. Others feeling she should receive the death penalty. It was a circus around the courthouse.

I lived in Phoenix at the time of the trial, it was unreal. The level of personal involvement some people took with this case was unbelievable. In the end the jury felt she should be held accountable for her actions but that she didn't deserve death based on mitigating factors, one being her mental disorder.

Ms. Arias isn't the only Borderline with stories of rage, maybe not as gruesome of stories but stories none the less. One woman I talked to told me a story of rage, confusion, and upset. At the age of 19 she found out that her partner of several years was cheating on her. Now, not all of us have been in this situation but the ones that have will tell you that this is a confusing situation for a person without a personality disorder, let alone one with one.

In this given situation said woman became so enraged, so hurt that she turned to violence. She grabbed a shotgun, shoved it into his eye so hard it blacked his it. She then proceeded to shoot the gun into the ceiling. Thank goodness it wasn't into his head.

On another occasion a woman was set off by an unknown trigger and snapped in front of her whole family. Shoving a knife to her throat, she swore she was going to end it all. She was completely out of it with rage and confusion. As a trickle of blood ran down her neck she had no care or acknowledgment for her crying children or her parents standing in front of her. In the end, she ended up at the hospital for days, receiving the help that she so desperately needed.

In a much less extreme case, a woman was triggered by an unknown reason and proceeded to throw a large jar of unopened pickles at her husband's head. All the time screaming things that she later would not remember clear enough to repeat back. Luckily, her husband ducked in time. Becoming more enraged, by the fact she missed I am sure, she grabbed his coffee cup-throwing it at him. In the scuffle her finger was cut bad enough she had to receive stitches. The scar still reminds her of her instance of enragement.

Another extreme reaction to emotions I hear about is the extreme reaction to depression. Depression is defined by (Staff, n.d.) as "a persistent feeling of sadness and loss of interest. Also, called major depressive disorder or clinical depression, it affects how you feel, think and behave and can lead to a variety of emotional and physical problems. You may have trouble doing normal day-to-day activities. Sometimes you may feel as if life isn't worth living." Though this one I hear more of with Bipolar Disorder, I do hear about it from those diagnosed with BPD.

There are times when this sense of depression rips families apart. There are times when this depression destroys individuals from their core outwards. Times when it ultimately leaves the person a shell of the person the used to be. Sometimes this depression is so deep the person takes their own life.

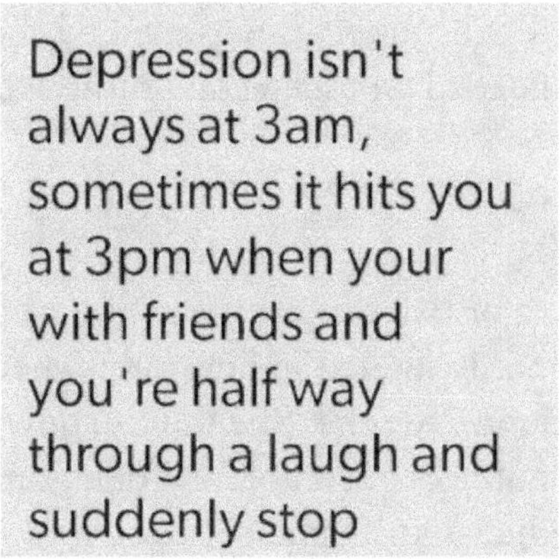

Depression isn't always at 3am, sometimes it hits you at 3pm when your with friends and you're half way through a laugh and suddenly stop

Figure 3 Picture Courtesy of Scream Poems

I have heard of women/men so depressed they lose their children to the state or to their soon to be ex-husband/ex-wives. All from being so unhappy in their home life they find themselves unable to function. One woman told of a time when her ex-boyfriend held a crossbow to her chest. She had him arrested as a result, In the mix of it all her child was left with her ex's parents. Whenever she tried to get her child back the police informed her that her child was fine where he was.

Being young at the time she let it be and left her child with her ex's parents, feeling he was safe where he was. After a month, her ex got out of jail and his parents released the child to him. He refused to let her see her child at all. Two weeks later she said that she received a summons in the court saying that she had to be in court at 8:30AM. That day they actually started court at 8AM and the woman ended up losing all custody of her child. Absolutely devastated by the events the woman needed an escape and turned to drugs.

I'm not talking one or two drugs either. She went at it full force and eventually landed in her room where she didn't leave for around 2 weeks. She didn't shower, barely ate. She was utterly miserable. At one point, she recounted how she had a knife and seriously contemplated suicide. At the end of her rope, childless, she felt as if she had no hope. In her head her child was better off without her and the world was better off without her too. An unexpected visit from a friend is all that saved her from an untimely death.

Another woman that I spoke to could tie her depression down to almost a schedule. She said that about every week and a half (before she got sober and started working) she would slip into deep bouts of depression. These were so bad that there were times that she refused to speak to even her husband or siblings for days-even weeks. She blamed herself for everything whenever she was like this. She even blamed herself for the rain.

She'd go a week or more without showering, changing her clothes, brushing her hair whenever she was depressed. She said that every couple of months it would get so bad that she wouldn't even get out of bed for 3-4 days straight. She got so sick of hearing everyone giving her a hard time over it that she started claiming that she was sick just to cope.

Through the mix of it all she was dropped from seven doctors and five therapists for missing appointments and not rescheduling. She often skipped rescheduling appointments due to the guilt that she felt from missing said appointments. Her extreme depression affected her family more than she'll ever understand but her recovery from depression has overjoyed them more. Other than extreme reactions to situations in life there may be other behaviors that seem a bit on the extreme side as well.

3

There may be unpredictable and impulsive behavior which might include excessive spending, promiscuity, gambling, drug or alcohol abuse, shoplifting, overeating (Richard J. Corelli, n.d.).

I have been guilty of all but gambling in my life. Along with this disorder there are also identity instabilities that present with misperceptions and insecurity about one's career choices, friendships, life goals and values, self-identity, and sexuality. There is a deep-seated feeling that one is flawed, defective, damaged or bad in some way, with a tendency to go to extremes in thinking, feeling or behavior. (Richard J. Corelli, n.d.)

There isn't a day that goes by that I don't feel like I'm not good enough. This feeling isn't exclusive to just myself. Thousands feel it every day. It's a feeling of being flawed from the start. Like your parents made a mistake when they kept you. That feeling goes all the way back to 3rd grade with me. I have spent many days harping on this "fact" and wondering why I am here.

This reaches to other areas of my life as well. Whenever I have episodes of explosive behavior it tends to lead to times of impulsive behaviors where my medications are concerned. If I have a bad day I instantly think that my medications are not working and in turn I tend to "freak out" about it. I'll either quit taking them or I'll go to my psychiatrist and insist that the medications aren't working. This often leads to rash and often harmful effects. There was one time in particular that I had a really bad blow out with my husband and decided that my mood stabilizer was not working. The very next day I made an appointment and went in with the intentions of my medications being changed. My psychiatrist obliged and my mood stabilizer was discontinued that night. Less than 2 days later I was admitted in the hospital under the diagnosis of withdrawal from the medication that I had just been taken off (Gabapentin).

Not only was I in withdrawal, my mood was a mess. I was drenched in sweat. I was so sick to my stomach that I was sure I was dying and was so dizzy that the thought of standing up repulsed to me; to say the least. My head pounded and my chest felt like there was a brick on it, my anxiety was through the roof. For half a day, my hands stayed contracted due to hyperventilating over and over again. It was terrifying. My oxygen saturation wasn't normal and one of the paramedics told me on the way to the hospital that I could die from it, that I needed to control my breathing. This, of course, didn't help me control my breathing at all. I was in bad shape.

I spent 3 days and 2 nights in the hospital, 1 full day of which I was sure I was dying. In the end, I was discharged back on the same dosage of Gabapentin and a very complicated tapering schedule for the medication. It lasted 6 weeks and took me down 300 mgs. at a time. I also left with a new understanding for myself.

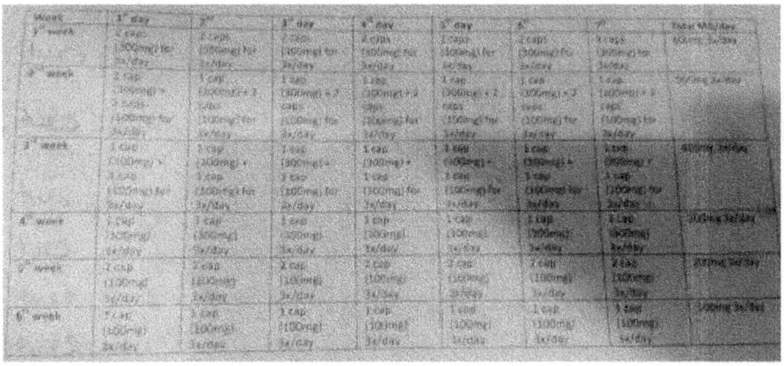

Figure 4 My Neurontin/Gabapentin taper schedule

I didn't feel 100 percent for about a week after I got out of the hospital. That first day back I honestly thought that I was going to have to go straight back to the hospital. My anxiety was so high that I thought that there was something wrong with my heart. I tried so hard to hold it together. In the end I succeeded beautifully.

My biggest issue with the whole situation was the wondering. Wondering if I should just stay on the medication at the dose I was on and leave it at that. Wondering if it was anxiety or my heart all the time. Wondering how I'd feel during the taper. This thought crossed my mind the most because I was so scared of how it felt to withdrawal off of it. Then in the back of my head I wondered if I can make this decision without making it impulsively. For the first time since my childhood I turned to faith for the answers. The whole thing was extremely stressful for me which in turn made my anxiety and stress even worse.

Another area of concern for people with BPD is extreme stress. In severe cases, there can be brief psychotic episodes with loss of contact with reality or bizarre behavior or symptoms. Even in less severe instances, there is often significant disruption of relationships and work performance. (Richard J. Corelli, n.d.) I know of a woman who was so sure her husband was cheating on her that she completely lost her mind. With her little children in the room she grabbed a knife threatening her husband. All the time yelling things that she had no recollection of saying in the aftermath.

The events of that night had to later be recounted to her as she cried out in terror at the fact that she was capable of it. Every word told to her increased her weeping. All she could think about was what her children must've thought.

There are women I have interviewed that cannot make it through a simple run to the store without it turning into a borderline break with reality. They start with the attitude towards their loved ones on the way for unknown reasons (mostly because they cannot remember what triggered them) and it ends with them barely making it through the store. When they finally arrive home they are so agitated from the trip things turn nuclear.

One husband told of a time like this with his wife. Once they returned home from the store she retreated to her room rather loudly. Upon entering the house she had said her piece she slammed the door so hard that she ripped the frame off. He said that he had no idea what she did that night in their room but she was asleep once he got to bed. She had no recollection of any of the events of that night the next morning. The night before she was psychotic, the next morning perfectly fine and chipper as can be. The only evidence left from that night was a broken T.V., the broken door, and deep self-inflicted scratches all over her arms.

I have also interviewed several people who have had multiple stays in the psych ward due to psychotic episodes. They tested positive for drugs they had no recollection of doing. There were times when nobody listens to them when they said this. Their cries of amnesia landed on deaf ears. It was written up as an excuse made by an addict when actually it was a truth told by a person suffering a mental break.

They really don't remember doing drugs and they really don't know how they got into their systems either. Most of the time they aren't saying the tests are wrong they are simply stating that they have no recollection of doing them. Honestly, they really should be listened too by the very people they are asking help from.

4

A pattern of intense and stormy relationships with family, friends, and loved ones, often veering from extreme closeness and love to extreme dislike or anger (Borderline Personality Disorder, n.d.) is another of the symptoms that affects me deeply.

I have spent my life balancing on the line between loving friends and loved ones and hating them. The feelings can sway from moment to moment and is greatly affected by my mood and their actions. The quickest way to change my affections from good to evil is to do something that I disapprove of. This black and white type of thinking is called "splitting."

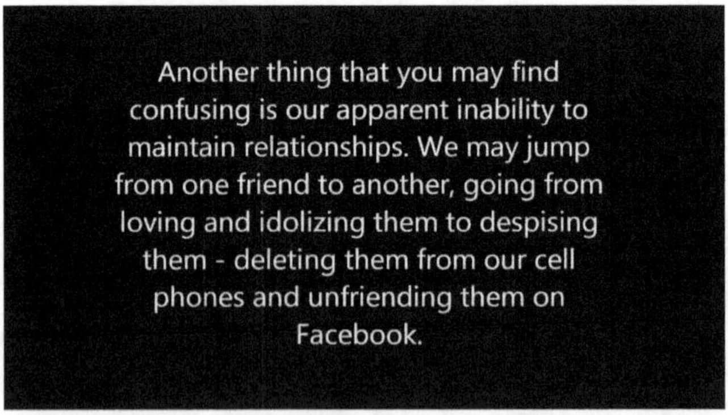

Another thing that you may find confusing is our apparent inability to maintain relationships. We may jump from one friend to another, going from loving and idolizing them to despising them - deleting them from our cell phones and unfriending them on Facebook.

Figure 5 Picture Courtesy of Google Images

You may not know what "splitting" is. Well, (Kristalyn Salters-Pedneault, What is Splitting, n.d.) explains it best whenever she says, "Splitting" is a term that describes difficulty with the ability to hold opposing thoughts, feelings, or beliefs about oneself or others. In other words, positive and negative attributes of a person are not joined together into a cohesive set of beliefs. "Splitting" is very common in people with Borderline Personality Disorder (BPD), and it leads people with BPD to view others and themselves in "all or nothing" terms. For example, a person with BPD may view one family member as always "good" and another as always "bad." Or, a person with BPD may see themselves as "good" one minute, but shift to seeing themselves as all "bad" or even evil the next."

This "black and white" type of thinking or "splitting" has been my downfall on many occasions. In one conversation, my opinion can change. People tend to be completely good or completely bad and this change in opinion can happen in a second. This is more of a problem whenever I am un-medicated, but none-the-less it is an issue. This happens with my siblings, friends, husband, just about everyone. Once you do one thing, maybe two, that I find messed up or that I find annoying-I am done. All it takes is one disappointment, one beyond annoying action and I begin erasing you from my life.

It is like the end of the earth to me. In that moment, you are all evil. Then in a second's notice something will change my mind and I love you again.

One girl I interviewed told of how rocky her and her husband's relationship is. She feels it is her fault due to her black and white thinking. She tries so hard not to snap whenever he does things that get to her but in her head things only work one way. As soon as he snaps back at her he becomes evil.

She starts with just getting a little snappy with him, every word flows with such disdain that it is next to unbelievable. Then he snaps back, in true smartass style. From there she claims that it always escalates because she always "splits" and he becomes evil to her. In the end the house could be destroyed, she may have punched, scratched, or bit him. Maybe even hurt herself. (This goes back to the intense rage and extreme reactions) At some point she sometimes becomes so angry that she completely shuts down emotionally- unable to feel anything. Per her this is a regular occurrence.

You see, by "shuts down" I mean that a large percentage of us can emotionally shut down whenever things become too much. This "black and white" thinking, or "splitting," leads to the ability to shut our emotions off in a second-without warning. We simply distance ourselves. This is a classic symptom of a

Borderline- the ability to shut down when things become too much. This symptom accompanied with the tendency to become angry also helps lead to patterns of intense and stormy relationships.

We get aggravated, then angry, then down right mean. We say things that hurt; do things that are hard to forget; possibly hurt ourselves or others; and then we shut down. Unless we have the most supportive partner, family member, or friend of course things are going to be stormy. Of course there are patterns of intensity in the relationships we hold. Only intense therapy, self-awareness, self-control, and possibly medications help us in our daily lives.

I'll give you a glimpse into my life through an example of this "black and white" thinking, or splitting. One day my husband came home with an attitude. I must add right off the bat that he had been coming home with an attitude for the last 2 years prior to this altercation due to stress at work. The last 3 months it had gotten out of control due to the stress of his friend moving in with us and working for my husband.

So, with that said, he came home and his attitude annoyed me almost right off the bat. We got into a small spat over his friend's medication price. A nonsense spat that meant nothing. I can say that now, then there is no way I would've admitted that, by this point in my mind- he was the enemy.

Not everything I do or say is a symptom of BPD.
I am allowed to have feelings.
I am allowed to have bad days.
I am allowed to make mistakes.
I am allowed to be impulsive.
I am allowed to be human.

Figure 6 Picture courtesy of BPD Pieces of Me

His attitude after that is what got to me. He commonly talks down to me; or I perceived him to talk down to me because that is how my mind works. To me any and everything said after a fight has to be said with attitude. I am aware that I do this but I am powerless to stop it. To me it seems that he gets snappy then says that he isn't. His saying that he isn't snapping, of course, must be said just to make the fight worse-not said in an effort to control the situation.

The thing is that he goes as far as to, sometimes, tell me that it is me and I need to speak to my therapist about "this." This is something that he chose to say during said argument on the day in question. This is something that I always snap over too. A "trigger" if you will.

I'm not always innocent in the words I say and this time I somewhat loudly pointed out that ever since his friend moved iin he has been mean (or I perceive him to have been being mean). Now saying this after we already have fought doesn't help the situation at all. Neither does the fact that I said this within earshot of his friend, which caused even bigger problems.

In the end, we were screaming at each other while closed up in our bathroom. Throwing daggers with our mouths and shooting bullets with our eyes we spoke to each other with disrespect on both sides. Who was more in the wrong is up for debate. It depends on who you speak to I suppose. I do know that if I had been able to stop the way I think and let things go the fight wouldn't have escalated into a round 2. If I didn't split and see him as all bad instead of him being a good person that is just disagreeing with me things would be a lot easier.

I will say that I do remember him asking me to see things from his point of view several times and not one time did I try to do so. Not once did I stop and give any validity to what he was feeling but I sure was demanding some validity for what I was feeling. I'll probably always feel as though he was in the wrong and what I did wasn't all that bad. Never stopping in the moment to hear or take account what his side was.

In fact, it seems to be a blur after the fact. I can't give too many exact accounts or quotes because I was so emotionally overwhelmed that I simply don't remember.

In the end I do remember one thing for sure-all I wanted was validity for my emotions and my feelings about the given situation. Did I act accordingly to receive the given validity I was seeking? Probably not. Does it matter now? Yes, because in the end we both got hurt thanks to my "black and white" thinking, or "splitting." in refusing to see both good and bad in my husband; in my refusal to stop, slow down, stop shouting, and see that there is another way to get my point across and that I have to think before I act we both got hurt.

Getting a handle on this disorder is a process and I am getting there. I am learning to have a relationship that is not stormy. Maybe learning how to do this will be a key to less depressed days in my life as well. Sadly, such a small thing escalated so quickly and became something so big.

This is all to normal in the life of most Borderlines. "I love you, I hate you" is a common thing with us. We think in "black and white" and love in those colors too.

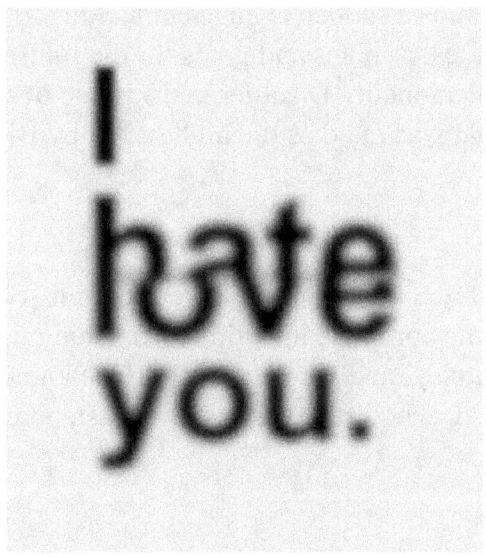

Figure 7 Picture Courtesy of Pinterest.com

5

Distorted and unstable self-image or sense of self, which can result in sudden changes in feelings, opinions, values, or plans and goals for the future (Borderline Personality Disorder, n.d.) is one of the symptoms that was rated as the highest felt by BPD sufferers.

I cannot tell you how many college programs I have started with the complete intention of finishing them. Life, time, money, and the fact that I do not know what I really want or who I really am is always standing in my way.

First, I wanted to be a heart surgeon. That was when I was straight out of high school. That quickly changed to a phlebotomist, then a medical assistant, then a medical transcriptionist, then a criminal justice major. I have bounced all over the board. I have no idea what I want to be. Who I want to be. That is a huge problem. That is a round block I cannot seem to step over or fit into that square hole called life. Something I cannot seem to fix, but desire so much to end. Something I suffer deeply with, but seldom think about. One of the silent pains of Borderline Personality Disorder.

People with BPD look
to others to provide
things they find
difficult to supply for
themselves, such as
self-esteem, approval,
and a sense of identity.

I often ask myself how one can succeed in life without a sense of self? How can you hold your head up high and walk the path to success if part of the time you truly hate yourself with every ounce of your being? How can you hold success in your hands if you can't grasp who you are? This is a problem that a lot of Borderlines must live with. A problem that many haven't figured out how to get past.

Do any of you have that one friend that seems to have had every job known to man, yet is still unhappy in their work? Maybe that friend is a Borderline suffering silently, trying to figure out who they are. Do any of you have that friend that has went to school for every major imaginable yet always drops out? Maybe you are witnessing a struggling Borderline sufferer.

This struggle often leads to a devaluation of self. We feel that there is something wrong with us and we will never find that spot we fit into. We feel out of place and thus feel unwanted in what we are doing. Many of us go to bed each night just hoping to figure out how to fit in when the actual problem is that we don't know who we are as people. Borderline Personality Disorder stole that sense of security from us. It stole our sense of self.

A big part of this unstable sense of self could be the high occurrence of child abuse reported from those diagnosed as Borderline. Forty to 76 percent of people with BPD report that they were sexually abused as children. 25 to 73 percent report that they were physically abused. (Kristalyn Salters-Pedneault, The Relationship Between Child Abuse and BPD, 2014) How can you be sure of who you are if you are broken from the very start?

6

    Whenever I find someone that I share a common interest with, that I connect with, I tend to elevate them above the rest. In the process, I tend to ignore, or neglect any other relationships that I have. This is done repeatedly, without control, depending on who I currently am talking to or based on whoever has disappointed me the most.

    I do not do this on purpose. It is almost an attention thing. I just do not have the attention span or patience to have more than 2 or 3 individuals that are close to me to begin with. When you mix that with the tendency to favor people things get tricky. The thing is that while I am doing this I am completely unaware that I am doing so. It never even occurs to me that I am neglecting my other relationships until it is too late. It is like I just expect that people will still be there whenever I get back around to checking in on them. I have lost many friendships because by the time I switch back to the person and realize that I have neglected the relationship the person wants nothing to do with me.

    It hurts when this happens but I have gotten used to it. This is a common occurrence with people diagnosed with Borderline Personality Disorder. When polling support groups, this came up often. People spoke of losing family members and friends due to inattention to the relationship, neglect. They spoke of how much it hurt and how much they wish they could change the way they do this. They wish they could get the lost relationships back.

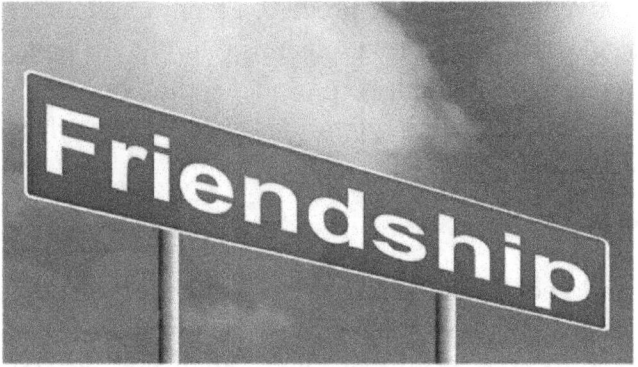

Figure 9 Picture Courtesy of Google Images

7

Anxiety is such a nasty condition. In fact, it affects up to 90 percent of people that are diagnosed with BPD and is brought on, typically, by times of stress. (Robert O. Friedel, n.d.)

Over the winter of 2015 I was stricken with my first real panic attack. I had never felt anything like it before in my life. My brother had often complained about having them and I always made light of it. Which was my ignorance shining through. These things are no joke. I feel mine in my stomach and chest; they come with a mix of sweaty palms, trembling, the fear of dying, and hot flashes. Sometimes I seriously think it is my heart and I need to go to the hospital.

Panic attacks are characterized by a discrete period of "intense fear" in which four or more of the following symptoms develop abruptly and reach a peak within 10 minutes:

-Palpitations

-Pounding heart, or increased heart rate

-Sweating

-Trembling or shaking

-Sensations of shortness of breath or smothering

-Feeling of choking

-Chest pain or discomfort

-Nausea or abdominal distress

-Feeling dizzy, unsteady, lightheaded, or faint

-Feelings of unreality or being detached from oneself

-Fear of losing control or going crazy

-Fear of dying

-Numbness or tingling sensations

-Chills or hot flashes (Robert O. Friedel, n.d.)

Normally to treat anxiety therapist use a class of medications called benzodiazepines. These medications are:

-Ativan (lorazepam)

-Klonopin (clonazepam)

-Xanax (alprazolam)

-Valium (diazepam).

(Kristalyn Salters-Pedneault, Anti-Anxiety Medications for BPD, n.d.)

There are other ways to treat anxiety though.

One method used to treat anxiety is "grounding." My little sister was taught this by her therapist and taught it to me. In order to "ground" yourself you find five things to look at, four things to touch, three things to hear, two things to smell, and one thing to taste. This method has been a life saver to me on many occasions.

Another method of treating anxiety without medication is meditation. There are many different meditation videos available online to anyone that wants to use them. Youtube.com is the website that I use in order to meditate. Search "guided meditations" and find the right one for you.

8

Recurring suicidal behaviors or threats or self-harming behavior, such as cutting are extreme symptoms of BPD. (Borderline Personality Disorder, n.d.) This is a big one.

There are women and men out there that become so depressed over almost anything that they resort to cutting themselves in order to be sure that they can still feel. For some the urge to cut comes from less tragic events. They have no intention of killing themselves. That is not the goal. Often times when a Borderline cuts they just want to be sure that they still have feelings at all. We realize how hard that is for other people to fathom.

Whenever you have such a degree of separation from your emotions yet at the same time live with your emotions on your sleeve what you feel sometimes becomes blurred. There are even times when we feel everything and nothing at the same time. It becomes too much to handle; too much to understand. In the mix of it all we cut in order to feel something at all.

On the other extreme, there are some people that feel so deeply they cut in order to relieve some of the feelings. The pain of the cut is felt as relief, not pain.

Borderlines are the patients psychologists fear most. As many as 75% hurt themselves, and approximately 10% commit suicide - an extraordinarily high suicide rate (by comparison, the suicide rate for mood disorders is about 6%). Borderline patients seem to have no internal governor; they are capable of deep love and profound rage almost simultaneously. They are powerfully connected to the people close to them and terrified by the possibility of losing them - yet attack those people so unexpectedly that they often ensure the very abandonment they fear. When they want to hold, they claw instead. Many therapists have no clue how to treat borderlines. And yet diagnosis of the condition appears to be on the rise.

Figure 10 Picture Courtesy of Pinterest.com

Suicide is a big issue with Borderlines. Up near 8 to 10 percent commit suicide despite receiving treatment. (Kristalyn Salters-Pedneault, Suicidality in Borderline Personality Disorder, n.d.) Not every person with Borderline Personality Disorder is suicidal or has suicidal tendencies. That is not what I am saying. The fact is that 8 to 10 percent is more than 50 percent higher than the suicide rate in the general population. (Kristalyn Salters-Pedneault, Suicidality in Borderline Personality Disorder, n.d.)

The fact is that the awareness for suicide is much higher with bipolar disorder even though the statistics show that 25 to 50 percent of people with Bipolar disorder attempt suicide in their lives (Caruso, n.d.) yet statistically 70 percent of people with BPD have at least one suicide attempt in their life. (Kristalyn Salters-Pedneault, Suicidality in Borderline Personality Disorder, n.d.) That is a giant jump in numbers without a massive jump in awareness.

This monster inside of us is quiet and potentially deadly. It deserves respect and awareness. It calls for it. It deserves it. 70 percent is a large number that cannot and should not be ignored. 8 to 10 percent success rate for suicide is gigantic. The pain that comes along with BPD is real and extremely deep. It can leave people feeling as if there is no way out. Their tendency to act impulsively also adds to the danger of potential suicide.

If you are suicidal or believe a loved one is you should call 911 immediately. Ask for said person to be taken to the emergency room for treatment. If you are not in urgent danger of suicide but are thinking about suicide, please contact the National Suicide Prevention Lifeline at 1-800-273-TALK.

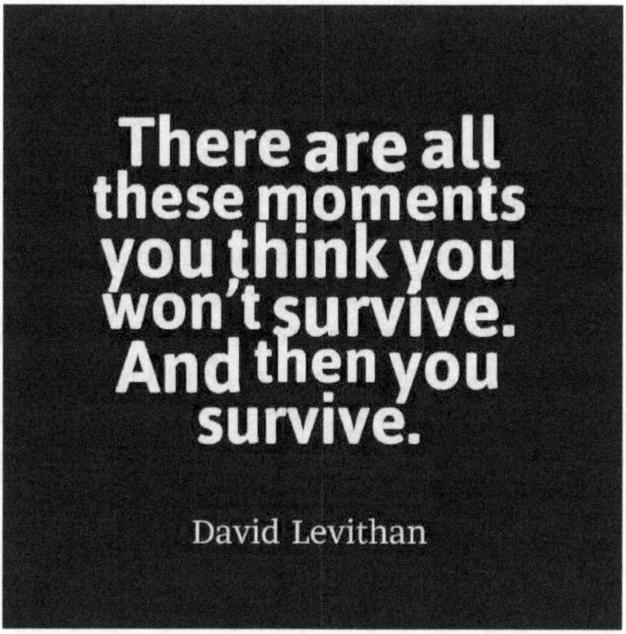

There are all
these moments
you think you
won't survive.
And then you
survive.

David Levithan

Figure 11 Picture Courtesy of Google Images

9

While many potentially bad points of having Borderline Personality Disorder have been brought to light throughout this book there are many good points to having BPD too. I'd like to end this book talking about them. From some points of view, the good definitely outweigh the bad points of this disorder. One good point being that intense feeling of emotions often fuel work success, not always confuse it. This intensity of emotions also often fuels the creative side of us. Many people with BPD are extremely artistic.

In addition to this, individuals with BPD often are people with above average intelligence. We are also often very caring people. Wearing your emotions on your sleeve can and will sometimes do that to a person. Throughout life the intensity of this disorder can lessen through therapy and self-realization. This is something to always hold on to. Something to value. We can and do get better. It takes a lot of work but it is possible. "Many BPD patients eventually make modest and even splendid recoveries." (On Good Authority, n.d.)

Borderline Personality Disorder sufferers also tend to be very trusting, very good friends. Whenever we make a new friend we are inclined to jump into the relationship with everything we have. The fact that we have issues connecting with people is what mostly leads us to do this. If you treat us right we will give you a lifelong friendship, a good-valuable friendship. We are also some of the best spouses. We give our marriages all we must give them as long as the person treats us right in return. We are kind and respectful people if we are receiving the kindness and respect back.

Parenting can be a struggle for BPD sufferers but those of us that can parent our children tend to be great parents. There are of course exceptions to this but for the most part it is the truth. We are patient with our children, as much as any parent can be. We are loving and more inclined to apologize for our actions because we don't want our children to feel bad about themselves for any reason. The way we often feel badly about ourselves. We also raise some of the best children into adulthood. Again, there are exceptions to this, but for the most part this tends to be the truth.

Being Borderline isn't all bad. There are even famous people that have either confirmed or are speculated as to having BPD. These people include, but are not limited to:

-Amy Winehouse

-Britney Spears

-Courtney Love

-Angelina Jolie-Pitt

-Lindsay Lohan per (Gluck, n.d.)

-Zelda Sayre Fitzgerald (writer F. Scott Fitzgerald's wife)

-Princess Diana

-Marilyn Monroe (Munson, n.d.).

You see, while BPD can be a nightmare it can also be a blessing. I am slowly learning this, others are as well. You must learn to take the bad with the good and smile whenever possible. You must learn to trust yourself and your therapist. You must learn to live your life to the fullest and love the people in your life that love you, without splitting on them. You must learn to identify your triggers and avoid them. You can and will survive this.

In the famous words of Mr. John Lennon,

"Everything will be okay in the end. If it's not okay, it's not the end."

Bibliography

Association, A. P. (2013). *Personality Disorders*. Retrieved from American Psychiatic Association DSM-V Development: http://www.dsm5.org/Documents/Personality%20Disor ders%20Fact%20Sheet.pdf

Borderline Personality Disorder. (n.d.). Retrieved from National Institutes of Mental Health: http://www.nimh.nih.gov/health/topics/Borderline-personality-disorder/index.shtml#part_145386

Caruso, K. (n.d.). *Bipolar DIsorder and Suicide*. Retrieved from suicide.org: http://www.suicide.org/bipolar-disorder-and-suicide.html

Gluck, S. (n.d.). *Famous People with Borderline Personality Disorder*. Retrieved from Healthy Place: http://www.healthyplace.com/personality-disorders/Borderline-personality-disorder/famous-people-with-Borderline-personality-disorder/

Korkeila J, K. L. (2015). *[Update on Current Care Guideline: Borderline Personality Disorder]*. Retrieved from US National Library of Medicine National Institutes of Health: http://www.ncbi.nlm.nih.gov/pubmed/26485941

Kristalyn Salters-Pedneault, P. (2014, June 16). *The Relationship Between Child Abuse and BPD*. Retrieved from abouthealth: http://BPD.about.com/od/causesofBPD/a/Abuse_ar.ht m

Kristalyn Salters-Pedneault, P. (n.d.). *Anti-Anxiety Medications for BPD*. Retrieved from abouthealth:

http://BPD.about.com/od/treatments/a/antianxiety.ht
m

Kristalyn Salters-Pedneault, P. (n.d.). *Suicidality in Borderline
Personality Disorder*. Retrieved from abouthealth:
http://BPD.about.com/od/understandingBPD/a/suicide
_ar.htm

Kristalyn Salters-Pedneault, P. (n.d.). *What is Splitting*. Retrieved
from about health:
http://BPD.about.com/od/faqs/f/splitting.htm

Munson, L. (n.d.). *Famous People With Borderline Personality
Disorder*. Retrieved from ehow:
http://www.ehow.com/facts_4814956_famous-people-
Borderline-personality-disorder.html

On Good Authority. (n.d.). Retrieved from Borderline Personality
Disorders:
http://www.ongoodauthority.com/individual_catalog/8
6

Richard J. Corelli, M. (n.d.). *Borderline Personality Disorder*.
Retrieved from web.stanford.edu:
http://web.stanford.edu/~corelli/Borderline.html

Robert O. Friedel, M. (n.d.). *Anxiety and Panic Attack Symptoms
Co-Occurring with Borderline Disorder*. Retrieved from
Borderline Personality Disorder: Demystified:
http://www.BPDdemystified.com/what-is-BPD/co-
occuring-disorders/anxiety-and-panic-attack-symptoms-
co-occurring-with-Borderline-disorder

Staff, M. (n.d.). *Diseases and Conditions: Depression*. Retrieved
from MayoClinic: http://www.mayoclinic.org/diseases-
conditions/depression/basics/definition/con-20032977

Statistics about Borderline Personality Disorder. (2015, August 13). Retrieved from Right Diagnosis: http://www.rightdiagnosis.com/b/Borderline_personality_disorder/stats.htm